CITIZEN'S COMMUNITY HEALTH INITIATIVES

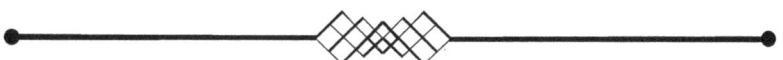

The Power of the People

FRANK OLIVER SALT

Copyright © 2020 by Frank Oliver Salt.

ISBN-978-1-6485-8207-3

All rights reserved. No part of this book may be reproduced or transmitted in any form or by any means, electronic or mechanical, including photocopying, recording, or by any information storage and retrieval system, without permission in writing from the copyright owner.

The views expressed in this work are solely those of the author and do not necessarily reflect the views of the publisher, and the publisher hereby disclaims any responsibility for them.

Matchstick Literary
1-888-306-8885
orders@matchliterary.com

Contents

Introduction vii
Acknowledgments xi

Chapter 1: The Challenge 1
Chapter 2: The Height and Breadth of Health of the Nation 4
Chapter 3: America, Citizens of a Republic:
            Can There Be Harmony? 8
Chapter 4: The Health of the Nation and its Population 14
Chapter 5: A Call to Action Concerning the Health Care Crisis 17
Chapter 6: Healthcare Reality from the Consumer Perspective 21
Chapter 7: Barriers and Potential Solutions to Citizen Action 25
Chapter 8: The Proposed Structure of the Working Organization 39
Chapter 9: The National Prison Dilemma:
            An Illustration of a Community Project 46
Chapter 10: Educational Initiatives 52
Chapter 11: The Role of Churches 58
Chapter 12: The Political Environment 60
Chapter 13: An Invitation 66
Chapter 14: The Part You Play 69

About the Author 71

Introduction

We are at a crossroad. The battle cry that helped to birth our nation is still relevant today. The wording may vary. The systems described have changed, but the sentiment is still the same. Tons of tea was dumped into the Boston Harbor because of taxation without representation. The people wanted a voice in the government, but that voice was being denied. So, the people had a party, the Boston Tea Party, rejecting a system that required their money but left them out of the planning and decision-making process.

Systems often develop over time, as needed, fueled by a variety of factors. As a result, periodically systems become unwieldy, stagnant, or out of control. The gears of operation get all gummed up. They seem to need new, fresh grease. The United States of America, operates with multiple, complex systems in place such as the medical system, the prison system, the educational system, and many other systems that might need a tune-up. These systems seldom evolve based on an overall strategic plan. Instead, they adapt to the demands and pressures of the environment and culture they are established to serve. In the human culture, they are established to serve us, the people.

A healthy nation requires healthy communities that develop and maintain effective systems. This requires the utilization of all available resources, careful strategic planning, and intentional, focused implementation. Unfortunately, the greatest resource, the human resource, which is abundantly available to every system, is underutilized. This book offers a way forward toward developing effective strategies to maximize human resources and to pave the way for meaningful representation in the systems that sustain us. This purpose will be accomplished through an organization called "Citizen's Community Health Initiatives". As the resourceful communities described in this book are established and maintained all across our land, they will surely help to improve health for the entire nation.

The medical, prison, educational, and other systems in America serve the people, and we, the people, appreciate what they do. However, as the professionals and appointees naturally take on more and more of the decisions and develop all the policies, the system becomes more mechanical and the people become objects of service instead of citizens with feelings, powers and rights. We must recognize that there are administrative and structural components that the population could be actively and legitimately questioning and modifying in each of these arenas.

The strategy outlined in this book calls for an association of representatives throughout the country to do the research, networking, and promotion necessary to effectively educate the public and implement a plan of action for the revitalization of any given system. May we, as a nation, encourage strategies that empower the people to utilize their talents, knowledge, and experience to enhance the health and vitality of the country. The power thus used by the people could drastically reduce systemic costs while increasing effectiveness.

The few projects suggested in this book by the author should be just to prime the pump. They could be regarded as starters, but dozens of even more significant and challenging problems will be welcomed from the fertile minds of you, who recognize and contemplate the neglected problems of our nation. The emphasis of "Citizen's Community Health Initiatives" will focus on social factors. We have to realize that citizens have much more freedom to explore and present ideas than appointees, elected officials or professionals have. Let's make good use of that freedom.

The approach to community action outlined on these pages could enhance any organization or system. The possible benefits have no limits. Please consider carefully as you contemplate these thoughts, how you might participate in this quiet revolution for the benefit of your country.

As government has grown and taken over more of the decision making, citizens have lost more of their independence, and let the government do it, whatever "it" is! It is time to recognize the fallacy of letting government have too much power, and to pick up our responsibilities of control of our lives, and of our futures.

The author.

Acknowledgments

I have been blessed with a family that has been very encouraging and patient with me through the years of this project's development.

My wife, Virginia, has been most patient and supportive through the years when we could have been enjoying much more of our sixty-five years together.

My son, Randy, and his wife, Arlene, have both made valuable contributions to this book's content. Arlene has spent many hours editing my several revisions, necessitated probably because of plowing new ground.

My son, Donovan, has patiently taken me through the computer-age entanglements of an old fellow from a different generation.

My friends, Steve and LeAnne Ebson, have also contributed important content and helped with editing and enriching, which I have very much appreciated.

At this time, I have exposed the book to only a few people to test their reaction. It has been very positive, indicating to me that they recognize the urgency, the need, and an opening for the people to exert their thinking power, and to take on a challenge that can mean a recovery of positive attitudes for this nation. Action by the people can take us beyond this present time of political gloom, squabble and dejection.

The writing of this book is only a beginning step. It is not just a book, but a plan of action that can go on and on. If the people catch a vision of what can be accomplished with this program, I will be so pleased and thank God for their vision.

If you are already involved up to your ears with great beneficial projects, please keep in mind that your awareness of this project strengthens the country, and is the first important step. Your wisdom comes from your ears up. You can share that at any time.

I am so thankful that you have invested your time with these thoughts. Thank you so much!

Your friend,
Frank Oliver Salt

Chapter One

The Challenge

America! "The land of the free and the home of the brave!"[1] We sing it in our national anthem. Saluting the American flag, we proclaim that we are "one nation, under God, indivisible, with liberty and justice for all."[2] Despite the challenges facing our country, this vision of freedom and courage; of liberty and justice, still flows energetically through our veins. We are still moved by the well-known ballad, penned to inspire the masses during the great depression; "This land is your land. This land is my land, from California to the New York Island, from the Redwood forest to the Gulf Stream waters, this land was made for you and me."[3]

If we were to truly embrace this land as our land, wouldn't it be a place where everyone has a voice, where each of us has a part to play? Yet, in a world seemingly swallowed up by huge government bureaucracies and giant, influential corporations; by complex, expensive medical systems and increasingly partisan politics, individual citizens are often left wondering what their part could possibly be. Is our single vote the limit of our ability to effect change? Does that single vote make any difference at all in the overall scheme of things? Where can we go to share our innovative ideas or utilize our skills and knowledge to help create a thriving, healthy populace? How can effective solutions, implemented in one part of the country, be shared and adapted to benefit communities throughout our great nation and the world? Our options seem limited, our voices silenced by the conglomerate complexity of it all.

In a world of multinational corporations controlling media mega-phones, it can seem like individual initiative no longer has a place. To come to this conclusion, however, would be to miss what the founding fathers of our nation understood so well. The conversations that change the world often start at the dining table and progress to the living room, the front porch, and the town hall. Liberty and justice for all is nothing if it does not continually spring from the heart of the individual citizen.

This book offers a way forward. It is an invitation to take back the conversation about our liberty and justice and place it where it still belongs: the dining room, the living room, the front porch, and the town hall. You are invited to follow in the footsteps of our founding fathers, to join groups of citizens who are excited by the challenge and power they can share from the depths of their own minds and hearts.

Dare to envision a system that works for all despite the financial and political pressures that threaten to make it otherwise. Dare to believe that you have an important contribution to make, that your voice can make a difference, and that your dreams for a better society can come true.

Through the simple yet profound approach to community action addressed in this book, every concerned citizen has an opportunity to effect change, to make the world a better place. By coming together with a determined unity of purpose, the citizens of The United States of America can raise their voices above partisan conflict and corporate special interests, above systemic decay and judicial entanglement, above bureaucratic obesity and fiscal mismanagement to truly experience the reality of being "One nation, under God, with liberty and justice for all."

1. *Key, Francis Scott, 1779-1843. "The Star-Spangled Banner." 1942: n. pag. Print.* (Scott)
2. *(4 USC Sec. 4)*
3. *Guthrie, Woody, 1940. This Land Is Your Land. Library of Congress,* pub 1945 (Guthrie)
4. *"The Pledge of Allegiance". Historic Documents. Independence Hall Association: ushistory.org. Retrieved 29 August 2012.*

Citizen's Notes

Chapter Two

The Height and Breadth of Health of the Nation

We are family. By DNA and by choice we are all connected with each other. When one of us is hurting, we are all affected. In the big picture, no one suffers alone. This fact can be as obvious as tax increases due to uninsured emergency room visits. It can be as subtle as one person's illness robbing the human race of his or her potential.

We must understand, for example, that the skyrocketing cost of medical care is not just a matter of out of control institutions. It may be the result of a myriad of choices that have become the seldom questioned norm of our generation. Just as no one person, profession, or group has created this problem, no single person, profession, or group can fix it. The same is true for an epidemic of diabetes. Diabetes is not just an individual problem to be treated with appropriate medication. It may be a development spawned by the collective choices of an entire generation. The chronic, systemic medical problems we face, as a country, do not affect the medical community alone. The masses are impacted, millions of people across the whole nation! Therefore, everyone has a right and a responsibility to participate in the search for solutions.

Our justice system is another example of our interconnectedness. We may assume that we have solved our problems by imprisoning those who have criminal convictions. Unfortunately, in my own community and all across our nation, new prisons and jails are being constructed because existing structures are bursting at the seams. Overcrowded correctional facilities affect us all in profound ways. People who have been put away, abandoned, forgotten, who no longer have a voice in even the minor details of their lives, can lose all hope of ever becoming productive members of society. This sense of futility can breed desperation and anger that festers and erupts into increased destruction and violence. And what of the creative contributions incarcerated people could offer if only their hope were restored, their voices heard?

Do we, the people, have any responsibility to work toward the restoration of these individuals back into healthy, productive involvement in society? How might our world be different if we saw each individual as a unique and valuable part of the whole, with a perspective no one else can offer? How might our justice system change if we, the people, were to actively invest in the lives of those trapped within it?

Our educational system is another example of our interconnectedness. We all understand that a child missing school could be a matter of the child's health, the parent's health, the child's classroom experience, bullying on the playground, or a combination of many factors. When a child gets discouraged and drops out of school, the whole community is impacted. School dropouts often turn to local gangs to find a sense of safety, identity and belonging. Could active community involvement in the school system make a difference? Could creative solutions discovered in one part of the country be adapted and implemented to benefit school children in another part of the country? Could our whole educational system be transformed by creative, innovative ideas that spring up as community members and educators come together to create a dynamic learning environment that no child would want to miss? The possibilities are limitless!

These examples illustrate how honest conversations about our interconnectedness are vital to the health and well-being of our nation. This book is an invitation to struggle together, as a community, with the big picture. We must come to the realization that it pays to make sure every person has a voice, even if we do not care about that person's situation or feelings. When those thought of as the least among us can contribute to the conversation as valued, respected members of the whole, we are all far more likely to work for the good of our communities. Furthermore, we may be delighted and surprised by the innovative ideas that are generated as we truly listen to and value each other.

Citizen's Notes

Chapter Three

America, Citizens of a Republic: Can There Be Harmony?

United we stand! Divided we fall. We are experiencing a great divide in our country that perhaps can be likened only to the civil war. Writing is difficult in these times because feelings are raw, and arguments run rampant! Statements often dramatically change meaning depending on who is quoting them. We must find ways to bring harmony to our organizations, to our country, and to our people. We must create new avenues through which we can communicate respectfully and effectively. Unless we start having better quality conversations, as a nation, we will self-destruct.

The United States has a strong foundation, grounded in the Constitution. This document has been revered for over two centuries. During the last few years, however, our Constitution has been challenged. There are those who desire to weaken the voice of the people in order to promote their own agenda. It has been said that big government makes small people. We, the people, need to keep that in mind, and step forward to energetically bolster the foundational principles outlined in our Constitution many years ago, to keep this country together and successful.

Unfortunately, we seem to be missing something; something that should bring us together! For whatever reason, we seem to have an aversion to involvement. Once we vote for our legislative representatives, we send them off to try to do the job without us. Thinking through the issues has been delegated. It is as if we assume a few people are knowledgeable and capable enough to solve all our problems for us. We have, for the most part, dropped out of the process of working together to develop new ideas and solve the problems our communities face. We must reclaim the right and responsibility of educating ourselves and working for the betterment of our institutions and communities. We must delegate, to the government, only those powers authorized in our Constitution.

Our nation is a republic. A simple dictionary definition of republic includes: "A State in which supreme power is held by the people and their elected representatives, and which has an elected or nominated president rather than a monarch." ("Republic." OxfordDictionaries.com. 2018. Web. Apr 5. 2018) This definition is in the spirit of what the founding fathers of this nation had in mind when they hammered out our constitution many years ago. This is the same document that has worked so well for us since the founding of this nation. It is the proven foundational document that most of the citizenry is determined to maintain as the best design to return this country back to its historical success.

What is required to return this nation to its destiny and capabilities? The same type of self-determination and stamina that was exhibited over two centuries ago. The people of the eighteenth and nineteenth centuries worked hard to develop a system of government that gave the people a voice. The same powers of mind and muscle must be applied in our generation so that we can reclaim that voice. Too many of the systems that sustain us have emerged and developed over time with little influence from the people these systems were intended to serve. It is vitally important that we, the people, move forward boldly, with integrity and determination, to initiate and propagate a broad-based platform upon which we, the people, work together to build healthy, vibrant communities. Hopefully, as we consider the ways in which the world is destroying itself, we will awaken to the seriousness of our times and take action!

Many of our nations' leaders are expressing concern about the dissension in the country, especially in the arenas of political and spiritual integrity. Too few of the leaders and citizens seem to recognize the joint nature of the responsibilities they share. Electing our leaders is only the beginning of our involvement. There has been a tendency for our leaders, once elected, to take full responsibilities upon themselves. That condition has been necessitated because of the weakness of the people. The expectation that citizens will lead with their thinking seems to have vanished. The result is, citizens abandon the needs that the nation has for their talents.

When running for elective office, most aspiring leaders imply that they want to respond to the wishes of the electorate. However, what channels can our leaders currently tap into to discover what people really want? For that matter, how do the people themselves arrive at a well-informed awareness of what is needed? Living in a republic implies that people and their thoughts count. Living in a constitutional republic requires our political leaders to respect the limits of power given them by the constitution. How can quality communication between the people and our elected leadership be achieved?

The challenge is to find a broad base of the US population who are prepared to participate intelligently in the creation of a new paradigm. Many professionals may be prepared to offer constructive participation. However, there must be enough lay participation to prevent professionals from distorting the counsel in favor of their own professions. While these people also deserve an ear to the top, they already have their association connections and the tremendous financial backing that often accompanies it. But I am advocating for the millions of intelligent citizens who have failed to recognize ownership of an effective voice. The form of constructive participation offered herein also provides access to the public for leaders, who currently have only a blurred avenue into the thinking and expertise of the population.

The effectiveness, even of the President himself, is limited by lack of access to the common-sense of ordinary people. He lives and works in an ivory tower with information filtered by aggressive lobbying, political maneuvering, media biases, marketing and propaganda machines, etc. How does the president gain access to the dependable talents of the populace?

The political processes themselves, at all levels, are sometimes tainted by discrepancies and back door deals. Is there really any way that all this hype could truly represent the wishes of the majority of American people? How can intelligent and thoughtful citizens, who are saddened and dismayed about what goes on in our country, reach out to devoted leaders, even political leaders, to encourage them and work with them in thought and process so the nation can become energized?

As evidenced by the 2016 election, the United States is grossly divided, with dangerous potential consequences. The people are frustrated beyond patience because legislative and government agencies seem to have no power to cope with the obvious problems and no mechanism to really deal with the growing anger of the people.

The real default lies at our doorsteps, dear citizens of this country. Without even realizing it, we have gradually lost our power through apathetic consent to governmental coddling and takeover. We have failed to exercise our prerogative to maintain some control of our systems and our lives. It will require much time and patience for determined citizens to recover the power of the people that has been forfeited through the years.

There is one major barrier to overcoming the stifling of the spirit of the people. Currently there is no mechanism in place, that I know of, to foster the generation, investigation and promotion of ideas for the improvement of our society. There must also be a process for testing, presenting and implementing ideas. As we have seen, political pressure cannot replace the participation of the people in the systems that sustain us. Without that participation, we are left wondering if we even have a voice. Current conditions of contention have grown beyond anyone's anticipation. There is certainly no need to imply fault for this dilemma. However, the remedy needs to come from the citizens.

It is the intent of this book to encourage a grass roots movement of the people to apply our intuitive and cognitive abilities to the problems we face in our communities. As committed citizens work together to make a positive difference in our neighborhoods, avenues for involvement will open up, generating a sense of excitement and momentum. Successes realized will, in turn, benefit the whole community. Herein lies our greatest resource, our most brilliant hope!

Citizen's Notes

Chapter Four

The Health of the Nation and its Population

A broadening gulf seems to be developing between the government and the general population. Frequent clashes of opinion make working together difficult. Harmony and friendly collaboration seem almost nonexistent. Conflicting objectives tear at the fabric of cooperation between the government and the populace. There seems to be no system in place that would enable the government to recognize and utilize the power of the people. Nor do the people recognize the power that they could potentially wield, the power of voice, reasoning, persuasion, and the vote.

No one is talking about the power of the people, not even the people. Are we forgetting the struggles that gave us our power? Have we abdicated our constitutional right and responsibility to insist that every system that sustains us be fully represented by us? Unless the government and the people can deal truthfully and fairly with each other, the outcome could be forfeiture. But if the government, and the business community would join a good faith, nonbinding, cooperative effort that includes employee and community participants, then b*illions* of dollars and many lives might be saved.

Generally, the citizens of the USA, Canada and other democratic nations have recognized for centuries that the power of democracy has defined our strength and success. Without our individual freedom to think, invent, and innovate, our lives would be severely hampered, and the power of our country would be compromised. A recovery requires mental exertion on the part of the citizens; serious exertion! The benefits realized would be reflected in the health of the people and of the nation.

In recent years, it seems that the power of the people has been relegated to the privilege of voting. All too frequently, after casting our vote, we sit back and let a few representatives make the decisions, while we are expected to accept the results. When citizens have no opening for their voices to be heard, a sense of futility prevails. Without an organizational structure to work with and a sense of team strength and encouragement we have little incentive or ability to take beginning steps.

This book will open avenues for action. It will enable us to gain confidence in our own ability to effect change. To have compatible teams as local sounding boards should give us courage to express our ideas more broadly.

Each system the teams explore may have its own professional language that can be confusing to the uninitiated, but concerned, observer. It is vitally important that we not succumb to feelings of inadequacy or intimidation when addressing the professionals or leaders of the systems we are working with. We each have our own arenas of experience and expertise. An outsider, viewing the overall system, may find systemic solutions that eluded a professional focused on one component of the system. We can, with confidence, encourage and facilitate the sharing of crucial knowledge possessed by those working within the system while maintaining our own commitment to building bridges of understanding. This collaboration will help provide the keys necessary for effective change in an area of your concern.

In chapter one of the ancient Bible book of Isaiah, we read, "Come now, let us reason together, says the Lord". With respect to the conditions in the USA, this simple message is the key! As we utilize this crucial key, we will be taking the first steps toward our recovery. Respectfully reasoning together, listening to one another's perspective, and valuing the contribution each person brings to the table can bring us into harmony and success. With the good of humanity as the foundational principle upon which we build, our current systems can be transformed into effective instruments established for the good of all.

Citizen's Notes

Chapter Five

A Call to Action Concerning the Health Care Crisis

The evidence is mounting. The medical system in the United States of America is in serious crisis. Information readily available in the media demonstrates that current trends are not sustainable.

The people need to get involved. This does not mean that they need to interfere with the professional practice of medicine, but they do need to understand and maybe interfere with administrative aspects of the system. There are too many conflicts in the system between government and people, between information and practice, between reports of advances in medicine and results, between Pharmaceuticals and purchasers, and between all of them and the poor people of this land.

What is this crisis, and what makes it so serious? The cost of medical treatment is rising dramatically. Along with that disturbing fact, diseases that can often be prevented through lifestyle are becoming more and more prevalent among the American people. Diabetes robs victims of their vision, their sense of touch, and possibly even their life. Obesity, which often leads to diabetes and other preventable diseases, has reached epidemic proportions. Cancer eats away at our bodies, stealing friends and loved ones from us. Heart disease strikes down a multitude of unsuspecting victims, often with no warning and no second chance. Strokes, lung disease, cirrhosis of the liver… the list is long.

If we were to consider only the current cost of medical treatment and the inflation rate that goes with it, the numbers alone are cause for serious alarm. With inflation rates for medical treatment fluctuating wildly, we cannot depend on stable projections for studies to draw conclusions from. In this current medical climate, it is difficult to establish a statistical foundation for new concepts or ideas, much less a revision of our established, traditional system.

In the past, the federal government has been hesitant to take on major reform because of the exorbitant cost and because of the lack of a supporting consensus from the American public. Most Americans, including medical professionals, have serious misgivings about surrendering the management of the system to government, and so far, the people have no options or voice, except to opt out. It seems clear that effective reforms will not emerge from the medical system itself. If current trends continue, bureaucratic takeover will inevitably come by default.

There is a growing realization among Americans that, even though we are the owners of our medical system, since we fund it, we have never been allowed to sit in the driver's seat. As passengers, our worry is festering into ominous frustration and anger because each trip, for medical attention, is becoming so much more expensive.

This book is an urgent appeal to the American people to take responsibility for our own health habits and to take ownership of a medical system that is headed for disaster. An alarmed and determined American public must implement an imaginative, effective intervention. This does not imply a change in relationship between a patient and doctor, but it could require some patients to study deeper, to get better understanding of their own conditions, options and responsibilities.

After years of observation and cogitation, the road-map outlined on these pages has emerged to help pave the way for the American people to become involved in the study of our own conditions and habits in our community, and the related costs of health care. If the financial and operational aspects of the practice of medicine were searched systematically by teams of volunteers I am sure solutions would be discovered, and the people would become educated for better health and savings.

There will be an effort to establish such a group of practical minded volunteers in each Chapter that is established, because this area of research has such a great potential for success. Do you fit in this picture?

When this task-force has been in operation for a period of time, I believe many from the medical community will enjoy working with us. That will strengthen the effort, modify possible contentions, enrich the results, and enlarge the scope of our work. The depth and extent of this problem justifies serious attention. The people need to be involved.

This book is a challenge to you, dear reader, to become a part of the solution. Together, many minds can search for ways to rebuild public confidence in the integrity and viability of the health system. Together we can find ways to educate and support the members of our community to insure a thriving populace. Together we can be the solution.

Citizen's Notes

Chapter Six

Healthcare Reality from the Consumer Perspective

We are participants in a system that has set us up to fail. The trauma that results from our lack of economical and effective healthcare is not only physical; it extends to mental, financial, political, and social stress. The negative results of this trauma can go as deep as bankruptcy or as broad as life threatening conditions. These conditions, and more, are health conditions, and are subject to your review.

If we, the people, are truly the owners of our medical system, since we fund it, why is there so little real representation by the citizens? How can true representation become a reality? Granted, occasional attempts are made to draw the public into the system, but usually only for the purpose of funding some project, not for sharing their thinking power. When some organization or professional group wants to raise money to promote a specific project, a public support panel is often utilized, or volunteer groups may be called upon, but the administrative structure and purposes of the entity remain untouched by the public.

In public services administration, there must be some form of citizen input, planning and reporting. Without genuine participatory representation, and with adverse conditions such as rapid and excessive cost increases, the credibility of the system and its professionals will decline, causing the eventual crisis we are currently experiencing. Through the ACA (Affordable Care Act) the government has implemented drastic actions to revamp a medical system in distress. However, these efforts are often countered by economic power groups, each offering solutions that tend to manipulate advantages to their own purposes; instead of for the benefit of the general public. Under such conditions, which have been brewing for decades, opportunities that would allow for appropriate citizen participation have not been created, accepted or welcomed. Public opportunity or effort to participate has been virtually nonexistent.

It is urgent that representatives of the public analyze the system in order to determine in what capacity the public can actively participate in the conversation about meaningful health reform. It is time for everyone to recognize the principle that those who pay for a system are the true owners of that system and are logically the ones to make sure that their investment is used to its maximum beneficial use. It is time for the citizens of our country to speak out because the health system we own, but have little voice in, impacts our lives from conception to death, affecting the quality of life for everyone in our society.

Since the general population has been isolated from the administrative and political workings of the medical system, the public is unable to make knowledgeable judgments about the economics, efficiency and quality of care provided by these systems. This is true even when we are making decisions about our own personal health. Yet the masses are expected to vote intelligently concerning political and/or personal health issues that impact millions of people and may have an adverse effect on our personal and/or national economic survival.

The ongoing controversial process we are now experiencing regarding medical care (ACA etc.) is extremely important, not so much because of what it is achieving, but because of the effect it is having on the American people. The posturing and political maneuvering make it increasingly evident that the focus is on insurance premiums, technology, politics and other economics, rather than on the health and well-being of the citizens. This is stirring up the frustration and anger of the population

Unfortunately, this anger currently lacks directional focus, and therefore is less useful in affecting change than it could be. One of the main reasons for the frustration is that medical costs have skyrocketed far beyond other major components of the economy. The medical system seems to demand that if we want to live comfortably we must have their services, and so we must pay their fees regardless of our ability to pay.

Perhaps this message could be stated in a kinder way, but the alternatives are few and obscure. Present philosophies about the medical system puts the medical industry, insurance companies, and the government in dominant, commanding positions that leave the general population uneducated, and therefore voiceless, about matters of health and well-being.

Citizen's Notes

Chapter Seven

Barriers and Potential Solutions to Citizen Action

If we, the citizens of this country, are the owners of our medical system, why is there so little action on the part of the people to effect change? Why do we go on, year after year, allowing a cumbersome and ineffective system to drain our resources, encourage our poor health habits, and throw drugs at our symptoms without addressing the real causes of our health problems? This section will explore seven barriers that prevent the transformation of our lives and circumstances into a more acceptable environment.

The first barrier to finding effective solutions is that the public has, for the most part, surrendered ownership of health care matters to profiteers and politicians, insurance companies, and the medical system itself. Even though we, the American public are the ones financing the system, we have little or no voice as to how our money will be utilized or who will benefit from our investment. As medical costs spiral out of control, the government offers increasingly bureaucratic solutions to a problem that can only be solved by a determined and informed public who have actively and vigorously seized responsibility for their own health and well-being.

The law of unintended consequences is at play here. Most, if not all of us, learn this law when we are very young. Indeed, we often become acquainted with it at the same time we learned about the law of gravity. Climbing the rail of our crib seemed like a splendid way to gain access to the wider world. Unfortunately, our first experience may have included finding ourselves in a sobbing heap underneath the site of our great achievement.

As we grow older and become functional members of a wider community, subject to its rules, we find more and more of our activities, even very personal ones, dictated to us. The growth of life-constraining rules that dictate how we will provide for our needs did not happen overnight but were moved along by the afore mentioned law of unintended consequences.

As an example of this dynamic, at the end of World War II, employers began looking for a way to attract employees in a tight labor market, without sending much of the money to the government in the form of taxes on monetary income, which were high as a result of the spending required to fight a major war. The unintended consequence was that employers became the major provider of health care. Employers didn't understand the medical business, so they hired medical insurance companies to manage their plans. The unintended consequences? People became accustomed to someone other than themselves talking to their doctor about the care plan that would be used to heal them. They complained about it, but found themselves helplessly standing by as someone else, not even related to them, determined what medical procedures would be covered by the third party. Furthermore, those who didn't have an employer providing their medical insurance, found obtaining insurance on their own was increasingly more expensive as insurance companies effectively aided those who had insurance provided by their employer with far more purchasing power.

We can no longer afford to apathetically expect politicians and massive industries to carry the majority of the responsibility for implementing major reform. Multiple urgent issues, partisan pressure, misinformed constituency, and special interest groups play tug-of-war at every level. This often leaves politicians ineffective, fragmented and paralyzed in the face of desperately needed change.

Efforts have certainly been made to solve our health care dilemmas through politics and legislation. When President Clinton first took office, much time and energy was expended to put a health care reform bill in place. Though the goals of that effort were not realized at that time, it served to bring the crisis to the forefront, alerting Americans that the political battle over this crucial issue had just begun.

Later, when President Obama took office, the urgency of the crisis had risen to such a high pitch that a lengthy and cumbersome document was foisted upon the public and voted into law almost sight unseen. Though intended to bring reform to a system on the verge of collapse, "The Affordable Care Act," otherwise known as "Obama Care," has added countless new regulations and enormous financial complexity to a system already bogged down in political and financial mire. It seems that "Obama Care" has become another bureaucratic monstrosity like the income tax system; tremendously expensive, out of control, and requiring enormous administrative oversight. On top of that, the citizens of the United States are still suffering and dying from an epidemic of preventable diseases, with little awareness of the lifestyle choices that might lead to a vibrant, healthy populace.

We owe a debt of gratitude to President Obama for having the courage to bring the attention of the people so forcefully to the medical crisis we are in today. The implementation of "The Affordable Care Act," and the failure of Congress to repeal and replace it, despite a skinny Republican majority, has served to highlight the problems that have been building for half a century in the minds of the people themselves.

There is still at least one more mystery about the Affordable Care Act that has some people concerned. There were twenty-seven hundred pages in the original document, most of which few people know anything about. Rumor has it that the document grew to over ten thousand pages. What is in the ghost closet that could come out to plague us yet? How can the people have a voice in these matters?

A quiet revolution can be expected if intelligent people of integrity are willing to take on this most important challenge. This would be an army of volunteers, primarily, so as to eliminate politicization, profiteering, and favoritism. What an opportunity we would have, as fellow Americans, to replicate the spirit of selflessness which was demonstrated in the construction of the US Constitution. The objective of this citizen involvement could be a vital element to reducing the cost of medical care in the United States a large percent of the TRILLIONS it now costs us. If this was to happen, our nation would be among the best in the broad health measurements reported on by the World Health Organization instead of near the bottom of the list of nations.

The American public is becoming increasingly aware that we, as a nation, cannot continue in the direction we have been going. We can no longer afford to depend solely on bureaucratic solutions to secure our health and well-being as a nation.

Nor can we afford to depend on the medical care system itself to implement the meaningful reforms necessary for the needed revolution. The medical care industry has become so convoluted that no one part can bring about meaningful change. Each component of this industry is so enmeshed in interdependent patterns, that effective reform within the system itself is virtually impossible.

You and I, the citizens, must take on this daunting challenge. We must apply our minds and hearts to the task before us.

Through research, education and innovation, we must set aside our apathy and get involved in this quiet revolution for the health and well-being of our nation.

The second barrier to successful reformation is the concept that the government must be the generator and manager of change. In some situations, government intervention seems to be the only way a need can be met. At first glance, it would appear that primary government leadership is vital to the establishment of a national health program, especially in view of the haphazard growth of the medical industry over most of the last century. This, however, can be a dangerous assumption.

The danger of assuming that the government must take the initiative in order for change to occur is twofold. First, the government can tend to go too far with its control. Even seemingly good laws can be implemented that require a great deal of oversight, are difficult to enforce, and are not applicable in every situation. Moreover, even well-intentioned laws may infringe on the rights of the people.

The second danger of waiting on the government to initiate change is that the government tends to ignore the vast reservoir of knowledge and talent represented by the general population. It is easy for those in political leadership to bypass this resource because it is difficult to tap and because doing so may counter or jeopardize the ambitions of those in power.

The third barrier to resolution of the problems in our country is that politicians and citizens have been calling for reform, but there has been no satisfactory definition of what reform is. The term reform has been used so loosely that it may now be meaningless. With Obamacare, for instance, the main emphasis has been to force insurance companies to provide coverage for more of the population with the help of additional government backing, to shift financing mechanisms, and to write stiffer rules and regulations that include large penalties. This puts more of the system under government jurisdiction. The basis of the change is financial, legal, and penalty driven, not health improvement.

Maybe real reform would be to partner with the people, making available information that would help everyone understand what real health is and how to enjoy it with less expense and more knowledge. Community-based research programs that educate and support the local people in the pursuit and participation of healthy lifestyles is where the real savings can be realized. The government cannot achieve this unilaterally, especially when a large percentage of the population is against their program. Acceptance by the people must be by a strong majority in order to make it workable, acceptable, and effective.

True representatives of the people, who have open minds and hearts, with a purpose of promoting healthy living, could truly bring about a cultural revolution. With the support of the populace, in cooperation with local and federal governments and health care professionals, a health system can be established that will have the largest impact in modern times toward building a healthy society and a strong country.

The fourth barrier to finding solutions to the health care crisis is that the citizens of the United States have no official representation in the management of the confusing environment that is mistakenly labeled "Health Care". This is just a fact, not an indictment on any existing powers or individuals. There is no mechanism in place through which citizens can become meaningfully involved. It seems that the public is discouraged from investigating deeply into medical arenas, despite the fact that people live and die based on what goes on there.

In order for this barrier to be overcome, volunteer representatives of the public must be willing to explore health systems from neighboring communities, states, and countries around the world.

I will not venture further into speculation about what results might be expected in this area, but I am confident that when the people recognize that they are free to explore, and become knowledgeable, and have teams and partners to work with, they will find many ways to improve their lot. It is part of the process of the people finally getting a voice.

This sharing and caring process could potentially be the spark that brings unity of purpose to the concerned citizens of our country and around the world. The benefits are unlimited, extending in ever-broadening circles to everyone who receives care, to making the lives of the many dedicated professionals as pleasant and rewarding as possible, and finally to the satisfaction of the researchers who are putting it all together.

This systematic approach to community building offers a way forward. Citizens would be invited to submit questions to the teams, including subjects or ideas to explore and reports or conclusions on previous projects. Innovative groups already implementing community-based projects across the nation could join the "Citizen's Community Health Initiatives" network to spread the good news of their success, offer tips about the process, and expand their scope of influence. Legislators would have access to the thoughts and the power of the thinkers of our population. This access would create, for our elected leaders, a direct avenue to submit concerns to teams of citizens already organized to conduct needed research. The climax of this effort is that we, the people, would finally have a voice!

Efforts have usually taken the form of encouraging early medical diagnosis and treatment, which is a focus on symptoms. The government cannot accomplish such changes as are needed. Despite current political promises, politicians must work carefully with the structures and alliances to which they are now beholden. Likewise, medical care professionals cannot change the patterns of conformity that have been established through the decades without jeopardizing their credentialed relationships. You and I, the owners of the system, can and must initiate and promote the changes required for a health care revolution.

The Fifth barrier to finding solutions for this health system crisis is that there is no health care system in the United States. While the term "health care" is widely used in this country today, it is a misnomer. What we have is a medical system. In that system, practitioners focus mostly on remedial care, treating the symptoms of unhealthy people living unhealthy lifestyles. While most medical practitioners wish to encourage their patients toward healthy living, the structure of the medical system itself does not enable them to go very far in that direction. In a profit-oriented system that offers only illness related reimbursements, there is little incentive to vigorously promote healthy living.

To complicate matters even further, people entering the medical professions have been coached in a system that puts little emphasis on healthful living. I have read and heard that most doctors, when asked if there was a nutrition component to their education, will admit that it was almost nonexistent. I am told that most medical school text books are written and promoted by pharmaceutical companies. These companies are clearly more motivated toward selling their products than they are by prompting the kind of lifestyle that would make their products unnecessary.

Imagine what might happen in this country if citizens were challenged to find ways to counter customary thinking about medical care. What if people who are not already involved in the medical professions were to take on significant leadership roles within their communities in order to establish, through research, education, and innovation, a genuine system focused on healthy lifestyles?

In order for this quiet revolution to take place, the citizens of this country need to become involved. We must spearhead a revision of priorities, redefining the purpose of our efforts. By gathering as volunteers in our local communities we can determine how to work together to build a system that promotes a broader recognition of the many factors that contribute to vibrant health, both in the individual and in society.

I believe that most Medical Doctors will be very supportive of this kind of effort and program.

The sixth barrier to finding effective solutions is that politicians, health practitioners, researchers, financiers, and the citizens of this country are conditioned to think in terms of profit and loss, of power and economics. Illness feeds the system, requiring expensive treatments and medications. Diseases, that may be prevented through simple attitudes and lifestyle choices, are raging through our country at epidemic proportions.

The pressure that is building as a result of these life-threatening conditions seems to crowd out wellness. With so much emphasis on developing new medications, equipment, and procedures to relieve symptoms, preventive approaches are seldom mentioned. Therefore, the public has little understanding or concern for maintaining a healthy lifestyle.

Consider what might happen if a primary focus of our society was to educate the public about the basics of healthy living and provide the support systems necessary to help people maintain a healthy lifestyle. If our medical system was to emphasize the components required to insure lifelong vibrant health, with insurance companies offering incentives for healthy living, our current epidemic of preventable diseases could dramatically subside. The profit potential of effective preventive care is significantly lower than our current medical system allows. However, the benefits of a focus on promoting and maintaining healthy lifestyles might drastically reduce the cost of medical care to society and create an atmosphere of vitality and well-being.

In order for this health care revolution to take place, there must be a renewed interpretation of what preventive care truly is, not only among medical professionals, but also by a broad base of concerned citizens throughout the community. These citizens must actively take their place as leaders in evaluating, researching, implementing, and promoting positive health care alternatives, and discouraging those found to be damaging.

The seventh barrier to successful health reform is that no platform has been established to enable the public to participate in an overall assessment of the health environment through input and evaluation. It is the primary purpose of this book to set forth a broad-based platform, with a national scope, attractive and applicable to volunteers, to overcome these barriers. This platform would establish groups of morally disciplined citizens to speak for the true owners of the healthcare system in the United States. It starts locally, voluntarily, energetically, and develops a strong national influence, working in cooperation with legislators, the medical community, and the people.

The following chapter outlines the structure and function of the "Citizen's Community Health Initiatives", which will be initially established in Skagit County, Washington, where I live, if the people will pick up on this opportunity. I invite any other communities in the country to the challenge of being first, as long as the efforts are appropriately coordinated. From this careful beginning, from a rural county in Washington State, the fire should spread. The citizens of this nation will recognize the value of their voices, daring to envision and create a system that works for all by building on the platform of citizen initiation and participation.

> It is not the intent of this book or the author to question medical practices or the efficacy thereof! This is also not intended to question the medical educational process, the relationships within the medical field or the interactions between medical professionals and their patients.
>
> The concerns hereof are for the administrative, financial and social health of the country and its people, and for a viable, economical, and smoothly running health structure that reduces stress, fear and early death.

Frank Oliver Salt

Citizen's Notes

Chapter Eight

The Proposed Structure of the Working Organization

This section describes the structure and function of the Citizen's Community Health Initiatives. The initial pilot program, in Skagit County, Washington, is expected to be the first cellular Chapter of this organization. The purpose of this Chapter and all additional Chapters is to establish a think tank consisting of persons who have read the book "Citizens Community Health Initiatives," have been impressed that they should be involved and have the talent and the compulsion to serve their community in this way.

These Chapters will become an ever-broadening network of community-based teams who reach out to gather information and share ideas with other counties, governments, organizations or countries, as far as the interest reaches. In this fashion, knowledge can be garnered, great ideas can be shared, and solutions can be sought for the benefit of all humanity.

Each member of the chapter will be referred to as a Research Representative. The Chapter membership goal is for not more than one hundred Research Representatives. That allows for ten teams with an average of ten researchers per team; a manageable chapter size and configuration. Team size could be flexible within a seven to twenty-one range according to the complexity of the project. If the complement of one hundred researchers has been reached, and more help is needed, a pool of associates should be established, to provide special expertise, or to advance to permanent researcher status when those of the one hundred retire or withdraw.

Each applicant for the Research Representative position is considered on the basis of a written application, which allows for the applicant to suggest a project which he or she recommends to be researched, and explain why it is important. A request to join a specific team is also an important consideration. The request for the application form will be in the back of the book purchased or can be requested online from the organization headquarters at CitizensInitiatives@outlook.com

Since Skagit County has a population of about one hundred thousand people, one research representative per one thousand residents seems ideal for minimizing the burden while maximizing the representation. This ratio serves as a trial model for future chapters to be set up in other counties, or districts of appropriate size.

As time goes on, many projects will be replicated by chapters around the country to enrich the research by linking those teams of volunteers together. The necessary coordination and communication will be handled by the central office in Washington State.

A Chapter executive committee consisting of the Chapter Director and one appointed member of each research team, meets periodically by telephone, e-mail or in person to oversee the general operations of the Chapter. This includes making contacts, coordinating the research information, and discussing where and how the next steps are to be taken. This committee is responsible for considering the practicality of newly proposed projects, and determining what resources and support are necessary to insure the completion of ongoing projects in a timely manner. This committee is also responsible for communications; updating all committee members, the communities they serve, and other Chapters, as appropriate.

Each research team includes a leader and a leader's assistant. These positions are appointed by the Chief Executive Officer (CEO) and may be recommended by the team. Team leaders are responsible for planning each project, in cooperation with the CEO, projecting initial time frames and working with team members to determine specific job assignments. A given research team may be asked to carry on two or three separate projects over a period of time. Each team meets frequently enough to get an overview of progress and discuss strategy. A written summary is developed, which is then sent to each team member. As much as possible, meetings are conducted by telephone or e-mail.

As new members join the organization, they are encouraged to request a project according to their personal interest. Specific experience and expertise are also taken into consideration. Members may be asked to join a particular team where their skills or knowledge are especially needed, or to be a consultant for that team, as necessary. Team members may ask to be placed on a list for reassignment based on a special interest, a travel concern, or personal reasons. The organization strives to create an environment that is enjoyable, challenging and satisfying for the team members while securing beneficial outcomes for their community.

The Chapter CEO or assistant will meet with individual teams monthly to consider new ideas, and to obtain progress updates. Communication with the public must be maintained in order to tap into the wealth of wisdom and ideas available in the community. An important objective of this organization is to explore the strengths and weaknesses of our public, social, health, and educational systems for the purpose of keeping them balanced and effective. This is not to be imposing, but to provide connections, where useful, to fill in gaps, and to promote improvements and public confidence in systems and services.

The executive committee, consisting of the chairpersons from each team project and the executives, should meet monthly to consider requests that have been submitted or new potential projects. When a person from the community presents a project to be considered, that person should be entitled to join in the related presentation and discussion and may be considered for some level of further participation.

Much of the research of this organization focuses on discovering solutions that have been successfully implemented in other places. Team members are encouraged to initiate discussions with neighbors, friends, church members, club members, coworkers and family members in their search for ideas, as well as doing research on their own computers. This will likely stir interest throughout the community, bringing great ideas and important concerns to the surface. Thus, people will begin to realize that there are alternatives that could bring improvements. In this way, the people will be encouraged to feel their power and let it blossom.

When the research teams begin to sense positive movement in their ranks and see a spark of interest and excitement showing from the public, a movement is birthed! A whole country can begin to arise out of its lethargy! As we start to experience the hope and success of a people on the move, a resurgence seems inevitable. With our eyes thus opened, we can begin to take justice, power, and morality back into our own hands.

As team members of local chapters, are thus empowered, they collaborate regularly in order to share the results of their research with each other, to evaluate possible projects, and to offer comments, cautions, questions and/or suggestions.

Once consensus has been established that a proposal is feasible, beneficial, and achievable, the steps to implementation are initiated, starting with getting the approval and support of the public. Depending on the complexity of the project, it may need to be implemented in stages over a long period of time or with progressing objectives. The initial research team will remain involved throughout the project to ensure that the goals are met, and the intended benefits are achieved. Consultation with various professionals and others, who may have valuable input, is in order anywhere throughout the process.

Once a project has been successfully implemented and proven to be beneficial, it is indexed and posted for review by other chapters throughout the country. In this way, successful solutions are presented systematically and broadly.

The purpose of this system is to demonstrate that the people of this country have good minds and are willing to use their power to move this country beyond the vote.

By working to promote the overall wellbeing of the general population, the Citizen's Community Health Initiatives system offers hope and encouragement to each individual that their interests and concerns are being taken seriously, that the community is working together to find effective policies, procedures and solutions, and that each person's perspective is important to the process.

Citizen's Notes:
Possible Project Ideas

Chapter Nine

The National Prison Dilemma: An Illustration of a Community Project

The prison system is in crisis in the United States. Prisons and jails throughout our land are overcrowded. Inmates, released because they have served their time, often return shortly for committing a new crime. Overcrowding had become such a problem in Skagit County, Washington State, that a new jail has been constructed. This is a prominent concern in most cities, counties and federal facilities throughout our land. The United States incarcerates more people per capita than any other nation in the world. How long will it take for our new facilities to become overwhelmed again?

I believe that the majority of the administrative personnel in these institutions want to be progressive in their thinking and would do as much as possible to improve the chances of a prisoners' success upon release. The gap between officials work and aspirations, and the minds and lack of receptivity in the public sector may be hard to breach. But if public groups were to initiate exploratory studies and promote remedial actions I believe responses from all quarters would be surprisingly positive, especially if voluntary public participation was evident.

It could be that a change in the attitude of the public toward these institutions, and their residents, could enable amazing things to happen to our communities, to bring people together with amazing ideas, and enthusiasm.

I will leave the above thought here, and hope it matures, promoting active participation in the process of discovering some solutions.

The circumstances referred to are commonly recognized, extremely costly to the communities, and a worry to the public. Unfortunately, there is no organizational structure, at present, through which the public can become involved to complete much needed research or encourage officials of the system.

Envision with me a team of researchers taking on the issues of the jail system in their local community. They may wish to search the world for ways to reduce recidivism. They may have opportunity to collaborate with other teams from around the country with the same research project under way. Perhaps they are asking some very pertinent questions. Are there any successful approaches to reducing criminal activity and minimizing repeat offenses? Is there a good working relationship between prison officials and the public to cooperate in the successful coordination of or transition between incarceration and good living conditions? Is there a possible connection between diet and criminal behavior?

What program can we implement that will most effectively rehabilitate our restricted citizens, enabling them to recover their dignity, their peace of mind, and their potential to become accepted, healthy, productive members of society?

As you can see by considering only a few of the questions that need to be addressed, even if our elected officials and government employees were the most effective people on the planet, it would not be possible for them to do the amount of research necessary to find answers to these questions, much less to implement the solutions. However, teams of volunteers, committed to making a difference in their community, could collectively amass a large quantity of information, evaluate and adapt the most pertinent nuggets, and make proposals based on their informed enlightenment. Other teams around the county, working in coordination with the original research team, could share in the information, and we could go forward together.

What if the research team decided that a good way to reduce the jail population and rehabilitate its inmates is found in the book "Food & Behavior" by Barbara Reed Stitt. This book outlines a natural connection between criminal behavior and dietary habits. By simply changing their diet, Barbara watched over eighty percent of the people on probation, with whom she worked over a twelve-year period, become healthy, productive members of society. The following quote from her book suggests that there may be a satisfactory action to help relieve the problem of violence and crime in our nation.

"In this era of pervasive hopelessness about crime and delinquency, can there be any alternatives, any untried paths, which can possibly lead us out of this dark labyrinth of violence and fear? I believe there is such a path. It is a path along which I myself have traveled, along with thousands of probationers. Everyone who has stayed on the path has reached daylight, has never been in legal trouble again. Today they live normal, healthy, happy lives. And the first step down this path is the realization that a healthy body means a healthy mind."[1]

After researching a variety of programs that have been effective in reducing violence and crime, the team may decide that the Barbara Reed Stitt approach should be recommended to the prison authorities. Together, the team and prison officials would then explore how the system might benefit from more partnership between prison and community in the local jail and probation system. The next step would be for the team to explore various ways this program has been developed in settings similar to the local situation.

During this process the community representatives must concentrate on their own side of whatever new responsibilities they are entrusted with, and be cautious not to push ideas beyond the comfort zones of the prison management, professionals and community board members, who have years of experience in their present capacities. Cooperative relationships must be built and maintained. Rapport must be established. Confidences must be honored. That is why the chosen team leaders must be carefully selected and matched to such responsibilities.

With a project of this magnitude and importance the staffing could be augmented by a larger research complement and possibly special associates from the community who have an interest and ideas to contribute.

The payoff in the successful rehabilitation of individuals to lives of respect and dignity could be well worth the effort. This program can provide a rich recovery of the hope and potential of human beings. It also can be a source of pride and financial benefit for the community.

We cannot expect the Justice System to bear the expense of a rehabilitation program such as the one mentioned above, unless savings in human life and program expense can be demonstrated. However, if carefully chosen volunteers were appointed to visit and monitor the progress of prisoners, supporting, encouraging and partnering with them while they are incarcerated, a more successful re-entry to society for the cooperative prisoner should be expected. Programs that are now in place should be studied and cooperated with, or supplemented. The cost savings and benefits to the community and society may go way beyond what a regular jail system can normally do.

From the perspective of the prisoner, he or she has been abandoned by the community for a specified period, sequestered with others that may be incompatible, without normal control of life circumstances, and with very little prospect of improvement when released.

What does this have to do with the health of the community? Much in many ways. There are multiple aspects to health; physical, mental, spiritual, moral, relational, financial, familial, social and a broad spectrum beyond. The opportunities for prisoners to participate in programs to enhance their experiences, with the assistance of volunteers from the community, could change a hopeless prison hell into something beneficial for a lifetime. This benefit would extend, not only to the prison residents, but also to their families, the community, the economy, and many other arenas of society. Most important is the respect the cooperative former prisoner can gain.

[1.] Barbara Reed Stitt, *Food & Behavior*, (Natural Press), p. 135

Citizen's Notes:
Possible Project Ideas

Chapter Ten

Educational Initiatives

We are all connected. It takes a community to raise a child. Positive, joyful interactions are crucial to a child's health and wellbeing. Getting a well-rounded education must include effective communication skills, conflict resolution, and other tools required to build healthy, joyful relationships. A good education also prepares students for meaningful employment and active participation in the society they are immersed in.

Community support and encouragement for children and their families is needed now more than ever before. We live in a country where drug addiction is devastating family systems, and where abuse or neglect leaves children traumatized at a very young age. Children impacted by these social problems often grow up feeling isolated, alone in the world, and convinced that no one cares! These children are more likely to turn to drugs, crime, or violence in a misguided attempt to get their physical, social, or emotional needs met. These are the very children targeted by predators who do not have their best interest in mind. Too often, in or near the periphery of schools, we hear of the horrific specter of drug and human trafficking decimating communities. The police find it more and more difficult to cope with this growing scourge. Community education and support is required beyond what law enforcement agencies and schools are equipped or enabled to provide. It is important for the community to be actively supportive, but not intrusive, in the lives of our children, and their families, especially those at high risk.

In these serious times it is important for the people of the communities to organize to focus on enriching the lives of children and their families. We cannot leave that privilege and responsibility solely on the shoulders of our educational personnel. But how can this be done?

There is currently no broad-based platform in place, that I know of, to facilitate the sharing of successful initiatives.

The goal of this book is to offer a framework for establishing Community Initiative teams across our nation and to link thinking people together in purposeful relationships. To have a team of citizen volunteers who focus on education in a district could bring a sense of community to many who have felt their aloneness.

These teams would do the research necessary to generate, or discover and implement, programs for resolving relationship problems between teachers and families, schools and businesses, school and students, scheduling, and student safety, bullying, conflicts between schools and family faith issues, or morality concerns. There are many issues that intermediary teams as wide as the nation could concentrate research on. There are problem issues which a parent or teacher cannot resolve, but which a community team is able to handle. Students are often trapped in the middle of such conflicts. Unless resolved in a sensitive manner, a conflict could leave its miserable mark on a person for years. With such an independent negotiator, the possibilities are endless, the potential benefit to society beyond measure.

For the community-based educational research team there must be a carefully planned approach to the community. The team must become discreetly aware of enough of family relationships to the school, the teachers, the transportation problems, the scheduling problems, and medical concerns, so the team can understand the problems that families have in coping with school requirements.

The team must focus on the needs of the children, the ability of the families to meet the requirements of the school, and on the relationships between all parties, because if there are hang-ups in any of these areas, all have to be involved in working things out amicably. These relationships are most important.

After such a team is appointed there may be a period of time before it is called upon for its services. The fact that there is such a service available locally, with the backup of other like services across the country, is a matter of prestige for the community.

The educational research team would prepare by exploring what are the perceived problems the local schools are experiencing, and then make the same assessment from the community, including concerns of parents, teachers, children, community and the general public. This builds awareness of the community on what conditions are, before the team has to take on any controversial matters. The orientation process of the team members is building in the meantime, and continues through experience and every project undertaken. Experiences are shared with the National office, which becomes like a confidential library of real life teaching experiences for teams around the country.

As the educational team matures, there will be a natural shift of attention to a more progressive approach, which would involve the study of innovative ideas to provide more benefits for teachers, students and parents and/or communities. Each community should be proud of its school and its students, and they should be proud of their community.

Local school boards, administrators, and staff would have much to gain by welcoming an exploratory team willing to share problems and explore solutions in school systems, especially since these teams bring the community with them, and are unattached to any controlling power. Much could be accomplished if a team of volunteers with freedom of thought and a high level of moral integrity, can appeal to many of the thinkers in the community, and at the same time help the community prosper.

I am convinced that many in our population are willing to come alive through an active relationship with their school or other system, which requires careful action along with an overall vision as to how, when, and where this can be accomplished. That is why the structure described herein is so urgently needed to be applied to the problems of schools, as well as other components of our society. Along with broadly searching for successful ideas to recommend for our own system's betterment, we need to open avenues for parents and teachers to personally express their ideas and concerns, and to participate in open dialogue.

And beyond that, a central management structure can be developed to coordinate the building of Chapters in counties or districts with you and your team. This would include building a resource library and maintaining and disseminating the useful information that can be developed by the thousands of researchers and planners that can be generated from such devotion.

Our children and our schools are in danger, and people of talent need to come together to discover what is already happening, and what can be done to make things better. This book does not offer solutions. It offers a mechanism to build a community that will give our children our very best.

Citizen's Notes:
Possible Project Ideas

Chapter Eleven

The Role of Churches

Though religious influence throughout the United States is not as powerful as it once was in some segments of our population, it can't be denied that spirituality has been an important influence throughout man's history. Our faith communities have been around for a long time with many of them seeking their own answers to these perplexing questions. We need to include their members in our teams as we search for answers.

The USA is called a Christian nation, and the majority of citizens regard it as such. The underlying principles of faith and morality have brought stability and a sense of purpose to their communities. Congregations meet for regular services, share meals together, and have ample opportunity to gather around the dining table, the living room or the front porch to consider ways they can make a positive difference in their world.

"Citizen's Community Health Initiatives", as outlined in this book, offer people the opportunity to systematically and intentionally have a positive impact in their own town and beyond. Members of all creeds and denominations need to take this opportunity to become proactive in the research groups described in these pages. This will blend their efforts with all other members of the community, pulling people together into beneficial purposes. These initiatives also provide the opportunity for people of faith to encourage their fellow members to extend their community involvement as well.

Citizen's Notes:
Possible Project Ideas

Chapter Twelve

The Political Environment

The "Citizen's Community Health Initiatives" will not be dealing with political matters because it is intended to be organized as a non-profit entity. If there is pressure to get into political matters, the task must be turned over to another organization, one that can work in that field.

Cooperating with Government Agencies

So far, I have alluded to social considerations generally, and do not consider that our work will have any different relationship with the government than any other nonprofit entity has. The proposed teams could, however, apply their talents to bringing reconciliation with State or local government agencies, or through easing legislative pressures.

The work will be done through in-depth review of all aspects of complicated matters by hundreds or even thousands of team members throughout the country. These are citizens who accept the challenge and enjoyment of devoting some of their retirement hours or other valuable time to consider how parts of the population are affected by the decisions of government. Hopefully, the teams will be demonstrating how many of our current difficulties can be taken care of in local or state jurisdictions long before they become a federal concern. This must be a goal to strive for, even though it is only conjecture at this point. Any present turmoil of our current systems opens the door for citizens to focus attention on the overreach of government, and the damage that can cause.

The "Citizen's Community Health Initiatives" and all related Chapters of the organization must be nonpartisan with respect to what they are assigned to and with respect to their duties with this organization. They must remain separate from the multitude of political controversies that swirl around us daily. As a non-profit organization, political or partisan types of controversies must be avoided. This may be difficult but requires constant monitoring to maintain the emphasis on the improvements that are best for society.

The national election of 2016 shows us that our legislators desperately need a broader base of involvement of the people. Granted, some legislators seem more interested in political games than in determining what the people want and are trying to tell them. But many of our leaders would gratefully welcome active and informed involvement from the public to help them acquire the information needed to follow the wishes of their electorate.

With legislators fighting among themselves, and with confusion in the media, the people have lost confidence in both. Without a structured organization, they have very little chance to express their dissatisfaction's or to help find solutions.

With confusion among the people, and with the murky messages coming from elected representatives, the people are left with little foundation on which to build their case, if they can come up with one. If the people have a case to present, where are the avenues to present it? Are the voices of the people limited to the voting system alone?

Even our voting system robs us of our voice in many ways, because it is contorted by billions of dollars funneled in from entities attempting to twist the thinking of voters so the real benefits to the people are submerged. Very large organizations, corporations, unions, cartels and other entities can flood the legitimate voting channels with billions of dollars to win profiteering avenues that are beyond the means of legitimate voters and which the people cannot compete with or combat. This is unfair to our citizens. It might take a while, but honest people must prevail.

There are dozens of organizations that are fighting for honesty and integrity in government These groups are attempting to educate the people about what individuals can do to save the nation. Each of these entities may have thousands or even millions of supporters who give periodic contributions anywhere from only a few dollars up to a few hundred. These financially limited people are sacrificing to win integrity for our country against those mentioned above who are seeking to win jackpots for themselves.

These are not political matters and need not be fought on a political level. These are matters that affect the lives and success of every individual at the local level and should be tackled by citizens of integrity on their home turf. As effective strategies are implemented, the word can spread to local city, county, and state governments as well as the federal government. Thus, the people can demonstrate what is necessary from government to enable citizens to enjoy lives of freedom, usefulness and productivity, and to enjoy their share of the benefits of prosperity. To accomplish this requires a structured program in enough communities to show what the people can do. Where there is demonstrated successful action at the community level, we should expect governments to respond.

There are many thousands of people in the United States of America who hear the news or read the papers and see through the contradictions and shenanigans intended to take advantage of the people or the government. We may sigh and say, "What can I or any one person do about this?" True, the overall situation is intimidating, but I hope this book inspires YOU to tackle the challenges that may be ahead of you or a friend that you believe has the right talent. May you experience the joy of working with other team members, unleashing your brain to solve problems that seemed uncontrollable as you looked at them alone. May you see the light dawning for your community as you birth solutions that could help countless other communities like yours or even bless all of humanity.

What is required is first a mechanism with a plan, and then you, or your friend!

When local citizen groups have adopted a program through their research or design which has the blessing and backing of their community, and while the plan is being promoted and carefully implemented, the concept would be shared with other chapters throughout the country. If there are other similar plans emerging concurrently, concepts and successes can be compared so that the smoothest application and processes can be found. Before full application, any conflicts with laws or present practices must be reconciled or compromised.

If there are national considerations, it may be necessary to work with state or federal legislative bodies over periods of time to attain a broad awareness of the values that are involved. This is where citizens, community powers, national leaders, Presidents, and even financial gurus can merge their interests for the benefit of citizens and communities at all levels. Think about the power of a Nation that works in unity for the good of all.

Citizen's Notes:
Possible Project Ideas

Chapter 13

An Invitation

As this book has repeatedly pointed out, a healthy nation requires healthy communities that develop and maintain effective systems. Respectfully reasoning together, listening to one another's perspective, and valuing the contribution each person brings to the table can bring us into harmony with one another in ways heretofore unseen. With the good of humanity as the foundational principle upon which we build, our current inadequate systems can be transformed into effective instruments established for the good of all.

Though this book only addressed a few of the systems that sustain us, the approach to community action proposed herein could enhance any organization or system. The possible benefits have no limits.

We must assume that successful experiments abound that need to be rediscovered from around the country, and even out of our local facilities. This is the work of the research teams, for whatever project they are part of. Therefore, a carefully planned and organized community program, such as the "Citizen's Community Health Initiatives" must be in place to enable the wisdom of the people to be expressed.

Please consider carefully, dear reader, how you might participate in this quiet revolution for the benefit of your country. This is your opportunity to be an active part of the dynamic process of working with your fellow citizens, in the problem area that YOU bring to the table, or of one already in process.

Take the challenge to develop new ideas to solve the problems our communities face. You can be a vital part of this grass roots movement. As committed citizens, we can work together to make a positive difference in our neighborhoods or participate on a think tank for broader based problems. As the network of "Citizen's Community Health Initiatives" grows and expands, a sense of excitement and momentum will most certainly be generated. Successes realized will, in turn, benefit the whole community. Herein lies our greatest resource, our most brilliant hope! The POWER OF THE PEOPLE!

Frank Oliver Salt

Citizen's Notes:
Possible Project Ideas

Chapter 14

The Part You Play

There comes a time when we must shake loose of our lethargy, and as concerned citizens, move into action with our whole heart and mind, and the Spiritual help we have access to. You are invited to become part of the solution. When concerned citizens are joining together to study issues, make recommendations and participate in bringing our Citizens back into action, good things can happen for our country.

We would like to have your name, email address, Postal address, telephone number, and a brief statement of any concern you feel this program should address, and why.

Please take the first step by sending your contact information to the following address: I will return an application form to you and an outline of the process of membership.

By email (Preferred):
CitizensInitiatives@outlook.com

or

Citizen's Community Health Initiatives
P.O. Box 860
Sedro-Woolley, WA 98284-0860

Frank Oliver Salt

Citizen's Notes:
Possible Project Ideas

About the Author

Frank Oliver Salt

Born in Toronto, Ontario, Canada 1928
High School: Oshawa Collegiate and Vocational Institute
Bank Clerk – Two Years
Bachelor of Science in Business Administration:
    Walla Walla College, Walla Walla, WA 1953
Married September 1952 – Virginia Lee Salt
U.S. Army – Medical Equipment Repair Specialist III
    Madigan Army Hospital
University of WA, Seattle – Prep. for postgraduate
Medical College of Virginia:
    MHA Hospital Administration 1958
University of Virginia Hosp. and Porter Hosp.
    Denver: Administrative Resident 1958– 59
        Life Fellow FACHE
American College of HealthCare Executives

    St Lukes Hospital, Spokane, WA:
    Assistant Administrator: 4.5 years.
Shawnee Mission Medical Center, Kansas City.
    Administrator CEO: 9 years.
Self-employed: Salt's Business and Tax Service Inc.
Hospital Commissioner–Elected Position–12 years.

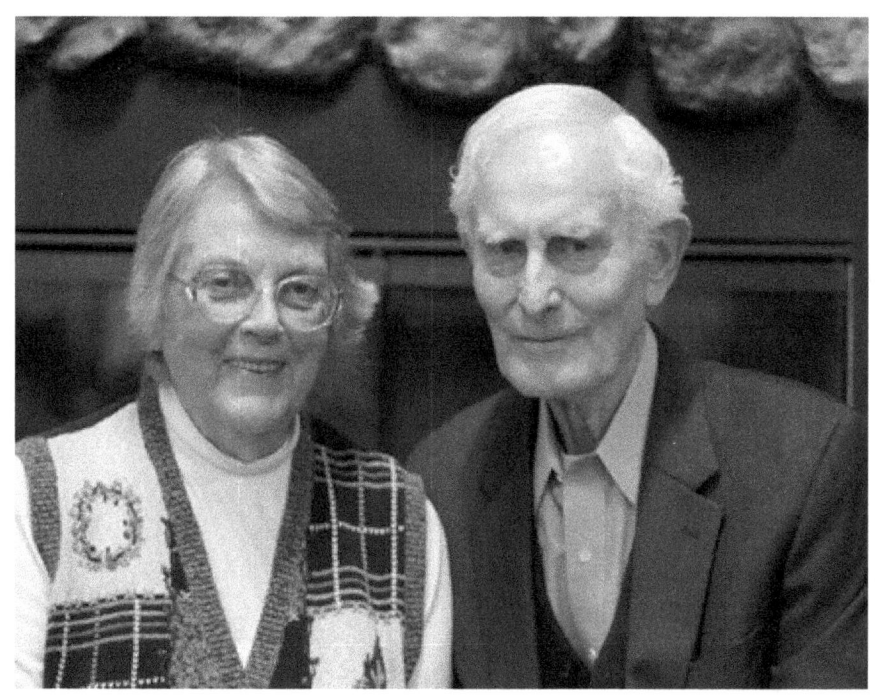

Author and founder Frank Oliver Salt, and wife Virginia Lee, photo taken at the recent celebration of their 65th wedding Anniversary.

www.ingramcontent.com/pod-product-compliance
Lightning Source LLC
Chambersburg PA
CBHW071120030426
42336CB00013BA/2152